An Insight into Menopause

See Through Reality and Know the facts about your Health.

Ila R. Wright.

Disclaimer

Copyright © by Ila R. Wright 2022. All rights reserved. Before this document is duplicated or reproduced in any manner, the publisher's consent must be gained. Therefore, the contents within can neither be stored electronically, transferred, nor kept in a database. Neither in part nor full can the document be copied, scanned, faxed, or retained without approval from the publisher or creator.

Table of contents

An Insight into Menopause

Disclaimer

Table of contents

Introduction

Chapter 1

Experiences associated with menopause.

Important facts

Chapter 2

Menopause Timing

Early and Untimely menopause.

Chapter 3

Menopause's revolutionary benefits

Chapter 4

Menopause's evolution

Complexities of menopause

Chapter 5

Hormone therapy

Chapter 6

Food plans for menopause

What constitutes a healthy menopause.

Variety of Foods to Eat

Conclusion

Introduction

At the point when a woman arrives at menopause, her feminine periods end for all time, and she is presently not able to become pregnant. Menopause is often alluded to as having happened when a woman has gone a year without having her period. A decrease in the ovaries' chemical production could likewise characterize it. Menopause isn't viewed as having occurred in women who have had a medical procedure to eliminate their uterus, yet at the same time have solid ovaries. Side effects typically begin to appear sooner after uterine expulsion. A woman's periods frequently become sporadic in the years paving the way to menopause, meaning they might endure longer or be more limited, or be lighter or heavier in how much of a stream there is. During this period, women frequently experience hot flashes, perspiration, or shivering. Four to five years can pass between hot glimmers. Other negative effects could include mood swings, difficulty sleeping, and a dry vagina. The severity of side effects varies among women. Early menopause is defined as the onset of menopause before the age of 45, and the untimely ovarian deficit is the term used to describe ovarian disappointment or the surgical evacuation of the ovaries before the age of 40. In addition to the side effects of menopause, which include hot flashes and streaks, night sweats, mood swings, arthralgia, and vaginal dryness, the actual effects of menopause also include bone loss, increased abdominal fat, unfavorable changes in a woman's cholesterol profile, and diminished vascular capacity. These changes put postmenopausal women at increased risk for osteoporosis, bone fracture, and cardio-metabolic infection (diabetes and cardiovascular sickness).

Menopause is typically a noticeable alteration. It has previously occurred in tobacco users. Other causes include chemotherapy of various kinds or a treatment that removes both ovaries. Menopause occurs physiologically as a result of a decrease in the production of the hormones progesterone and estrogen by the ovaries. Although not typically necessary, menopause's end can be confirmed by calculating the chemical concentrations in the urine or blood. Menopause is the opposite of menarche, the time when a woman's period first begins.

Side effects and the likelihood of bone misfortune are the key indicators for menopausal medication. Treatment may help with adverse effects. When it comes to hot flashes, it's commonly advised to avoid drinking alcohol, smoking, and consuming caffeine. You can also try lying down naked in a cold room and using a fan. Menopausal chemical therapy is the most effective treatment for menopausal side symptoms (MHT). Clonidine, gabapentin, or certain serotonin reuptake inhibitors are non-hormonal therapies for hot blazes. These won't cause side effects like joint pain or vaginal dryness, which affect more than 55% of women, to worsen. Exercise could help with sleep troubles. Many of the concerns concerning the application of MHT identified by more experienced studies are not typically viewed as obstacles to MHT in sound ladies. There isn't a lot of evidence to support the efficacy of elective medication. The use of phytoestrogens for diagnostic treatment is supported by preliminary research.

Chapter 1

Experiences associated with menopause.

Menopause knowledge can be traced back to the ancient Greeks. In reality, the term's roots may also be discovered in Greek: "men," which means month and is related to the word "moon," and "pauein," which denotes the need to pause or stop. The close of a woman's monthly (lunar) cycle, occurs at night. There is surprisingly little information about menopausal women from earlier eras, which is understandable given that life spans were shorter. It's estimated that in ancient Greece, at least 50% of women passed away by the age of 34. Additionally, the ancient population recognized that menopausal women were not the focus of much literature or research since it was believed that women were inferior to men and that a woman's value depended on her level of wealth. Menopause was thought of as a peculiar trait until around the eighteenth century, of that much we can be sure. In the 300 years that followed, mentalities changed and medical experts began to view the passage of life as a sickness. As a result, strange and unexpectedly dangerous remedies for menopause emerged.

By the Victorian era, menopause in particular, and women's reproductive health, in general, were the subjects of intense doubt. Doctors agreed that there was a link between the stomach and the mind that made all women more susceptible to mental illness. This was thought to be especially true for women going through menopause, who were acknowledged to suffer the negative effects of a condition known as "climacteric lunacy." So they decided that placing these women in shelters would be the major constant treatment.

The Victorians held that a woman's ovaries "were the seat of female pith" and that everything idealistic about women originated from them. Therefore, if the ovaries were sick or stopped functioning (as they do at menopause), a woman was not of sound mind. They agreed to remove the responsible organs. They agreed that this would make women more resigned, pleasant, and hardworking. Following this, many women had their ovaries carefully removed, a procedure that was thought to be crucial in treating mental illnesses like nymphomania and schizophrenia. Since women were designed to be mothers, any display of sexual longing was viewed as a sign of insanity. One London doctor went so far as to recommend clitoridectomy for these women, which entails carefully removing the clitoris. He was convinced that the system would prevent a woman from degenerating into incompetence. Before the century was out, the theory that menopause was caused by chemicals finally began to gain traction.

Ovarian chemicals were separated as clinical research developed and the workings of the endocrine framework were discovered, providing clinicians with a more logical perspective on menopause. The belief that menopause was a sign of hysteria gradually gave way to the idea that a woman's "lost womanliness" might be restored by pharmaceutical drugs. By that time, the pharmaceutical company Merck had developed a medication called Ovarian that entailed mixing powdered, pounded, and wilted cow ovaries. the ensuing medications. During the 1960s, the popularity of synthetic estrogen therapy was growing, but it would take a very long time for its long-term effects to be discovered. A study conducted in 2002 by the Ladies' Wellbeing Initiative (WHI) revealed that the combination of synthetic chemicals present in these therapies may increase a woman's risk for breast cancer, a heart attack at any time, and stroke. In any case, by 2004, a closer look at the review's findings led the WHI to claim that the threats described two years earlier might have been exaggerated. It is depressing to think that women from hundreds of years ago were viewed as insane at a time when they might sense the disruptive effects of changing chemicals. Fortunately, we have made significant progress in how we see menopause, its side effects, and medications in our daily lives. Never again is it anything to be afraid of, yet there comes a time in a woman's life when she can move forward with a sense of just having gained independence from the menstrual cycle, cramps, and unplanned pregnancy, and that's just the beginning. The fact that many women are still severely impacted by the menopausal side effects is something that hasn't altered throughout time. Bioidentical chemical medications are now providing relief. Bioidentical substances are initially not human, yet they resemble human substances in terms of capability and natural design. Bioidenticals are derived from plants like soybeans and wild sweet potatoes, and they mimic a material structure that is naturally occurring in a woman's body. Fewer side effects and more significant medicinal benefits are the results. The symptoms of menopause don't have to be painful for today's modern lady. The quality of life that every woman wants can be restored through hormone treatment (HT), which can assist in redressing imbalances.

Important facts

For women, menopause marks the end of their regenerative years and is one stage in a continuum of life stages. A woman cannot become pregnant after menopause, except in rare circumstances when specific ripening medications are used. Between the ages of 45 and 55, most women go through menopause, which is a typical aspect of organic aging. The inability of the ovary to produce follicles and a decline in blood estrogen levels cause menopause. Changes in the monthly cycle often signal the beginning of the menopausal process, which might be delayed. The term "perimenopause" refers to the period that begins when these symptoms are first observed and ends a year following the last period for women.

Perimenopause can last for a long time and affect one's physical, emotional, social, and spiritual well-being. Various hormonal and non-hormonal interventions can lessen the consequences of perimenopause. Menopause may result from surgery or care management.

How menopause occurs

Due to the reduction of ovarian follicular capacity, menopause typically occurs toward the end of the monthly feminine cycle, also known as a "period" or "female period." This suggests that the ovaries stopped producing eggs during treatment. The frequency and duration of the period vary depending on the hypothetical length of a woman's life; nonetheless, for most women worldwide, normal menopause occurs between the ages of 45 and 55. After 12 consecutive months without a feminine cycle, for which there could be no other obvious physiological or obsessional cause and without even a hint of therapeutic intervention, regular menopause is thought to have occurred. Several women go through menopause before turning 40 years old. This "untimely menopause" may be brought on by particular chromosomal anomalies, immune system problems, or other unidentified factors. Even though there are correlations between the age at menopause and specific demographic, health, and hereditary factors, it is impossible to predict when a single woman will experience menopause. Surgery that involves the removal of both ovaries or medical treatments that result in the loss of ovarian function can both cause the onset of menopause (for instance, radiation treatment or chemotherapy). Many women have previously stopped menstruating before menopause, including those who have undergone specific surgeries (such as a hysterectomy or the delicate removal of their uterine lining), as well as those who use specific hormonal contraceptives and other medications that cause infrequent or skipped periods.

Chapter 2

Menopause Timing

Your monthly menstrual cycles end with the onset of menopause. After a year has passed without feminine menstruation, it is examined. Menopause is a typical natural cycle. However, the actual side effects of menopause, such as hot flashes and severe side effects, may disturb your sleep, sap your vitality, or affect your comfort at home. From dietary changes to pharmacological therapy, there are several effective medications available.

Causes

Normally, diminishing regenerative chemicals can cause menopause. Your ovaries start producing less estrogen and progesterone, the hormones that control the female cycle, as you get closer to your late 30s and your ripeness decreases. Your periods may become heavier or lighter, more or less frequent, longer or less continuous, or stop altogether in your 40s. Typically, this happens around age 51, when your ovaries stop producing eggs.

an operation that removes the ovaries (oophorectomy). The hormones that regulate your menstruation, such as progesterone and estrogen, are produced by your ovaries. Menopause occurs quickly after having your ovaries removed by surgery. Your periods end, and you'll likely have hot flashes along with other menopausal symptoms and indicators. Because hormonal changes occur rapidly rather than gradually over a long period, signs and side effects can be severe.

• A hysterectomy, an operation that removes your uterus but leaves your ovaries intact, typically doesn't result in early menopause. Although you no longer have periods, your ovaries continue to release eggs and generate estrogen and progesterone.

Additionally, radiation therapy. These illness therapies have the potential to cause menopause, resulting in side effects such as hot flashes during or shortly after treatment. Following chemotherapy, the cessation of menstruation (and ripeness) isn't usually permanent, thus contraception may still be necessary. If radiation is directed at the ovaries, it may have an impact on ovarian capacity. Menopause is unaffected by radiation therapy administered to various body parts, such as the head and neck or tissue in the bosom.

• A lack of essential ovarian tissue. Menopause occurs in about 1% of women before age 40. (untimely menopause). Untimely menopause may be caused by your ovaries failing to produce the normal amounts of conceptive hormones (essential ovarian deficit), which can be caused by immune system disease or inherited factors. However, there is frequently no explanation for early menopause. Chemical therapy is frequently advised for these women, essentially up until the typical menopausal time, to protect the bones, heart, and brain.

Negative Effects

You may experience the following symptoms and warning indications in the months or years leading up to menopause (perimenopause):

Periodic sporadic

Fiery blazes

Chills

Sweats at night

Changes in mental state

Gaining weight and improving back digestion

Dry skin and thinning hair

loss of bosom completion

Signs and symptoms, as well as alterations to the menstrual cycle, can vary among women. Before your periods finish, you'll probably experience some oddities.

Period skips are expected and common during perimenopause. Female periods frequently skip a month and come back, or skip for a while and then resume monthly cycles for a few months. Periods also typically occur on shorter cycles, making them closer together. Although periods can be unexpected, pregnancy is possible. Consider a pregnancy test if you have skipped a period but are unaware that you have started the menopausal transition.

Early and Untimely menopause.

During menopause, you are no longer able to become pregnant. The typical woman or person assigned female at birth (AFAB) often experiences menopause in their mid-fifties. Before the age of 40, women and people with AFAB have untimely menopause, and before the age of 45, early menopause. These conditions have similar side effects to menopause as a whole, and the causes are frequently unknown.

Untimely menopause and early menopause are conditions in which a woman or person born into a female gender (AFAB) experiences menopause earlier than is often anticipated. When a woman's feminine periods stop, this is known as menopause. Menopause in healthy women often starts at age 51. Whenever you've gone 12 straight months without a period, you've gone through menopause.

Menopause isn't a cycle; rather, it's a particular moment when the period closes. When menopause starts before age 45, it is known as "early menopause."

When menopause starts before age 40, it is considered untimely.

What causes early and untimely menopause?

Large numbers of the reasons for untimely menopause can likewise be reasons for early menopause. A portion of these reasons incorporates malignant growth treatment, medical procedures, or certain medical issues. Be that as it may, in some cases, the reason is obscure. Anything that harms your ovaries or prevents your body from creating estrogen can cause menopause.

Early and untimely menopause likewise shares a significant number of similar side effects as menopause.

Some reasons for either an early or untimely menopause include:

Radiation or chemotherapy is used to treat illness.

An operation that removes your ovaries

Removal of your uterus by surgery (hysterectomy)

Early menopause in the family history

having your most memorable experience before the age of eleven

Chromosomal anomalies like Turner's syndrome or Delicate X.

illnesses of the immune system, such as thyroid disease, Crohn's disease, or rheumatoid arthritis.

Smoking tobacco.

ME/CFS stands for "myalgic encephalomyelitis/constant fatigue syndrome."

HIV-positive or Aids.

contaminants like measles

Sometimes there is no explanation for early or untimely menopause. In up to half of people, this is the case.

What are the side effects of early or untimely menopause?

Before your last period, you can start having erratic monthly cycles for a few years. Some of the most common signs of menopause include longer or shorter menstrual cycles, spotting in between periods, or changes in vaginal drainage. In the unlikely event that you go through erratic periods, speak with a medical services provider to look into possible causes. Many of the typical menopause side effects are present in various signs of untimely and early menopause. You might learn:

Migraines.

Fiery blazes.

Puffiness and discomfort in the vagina during intercourse

difficulty sleeping (sleep deprivation).

The successive urge to urinate.

additional recurrent urinary tract infections (UTIs).

additional recurrent urinary tract infections (UTIs). Either gaining or losing weight.

shrinking or going bald.

Significant alterations (crabbiness, temperament swings, melancholy, or tension).

Dry tongue, dry eyes, or dry skin

Bosom treat.

Energetic heart

The joint and muscular ache that throbs

Alterations to your sexual drive (charisma)

focusing on difficulties or becoming more careless.

What are the dangers of untimely or early menopause?

Individuals who go through menopause in their mid-30s will generally have more serious side effects of menopause. These side effects can prompt sexual brokenness or a loss of closeness. Furthermore, individuals who experience untimely or early menopause spend more years without the advantages of estrogen. Without commonplace measures of estrogen, you're at a more serious gamble for specific ailments like:

Osteoporosis.

Coronary disease.

Sadness.

Several neurological diseases exist, such as dementia and Parkinson's disease.

How to reduce the chance of experiencing early menopause

As far as you may be concerned, the majority of the causes of early menopause cannot be changed. The biggest lifestyle factor that could lead to early menopause is smoking. By giving up smoking, you can reduce your risk of experiencing menopause. In general, there are a variety of causes for menopause, such as medical conditions, treatments for illnesses, or medical issues.

Chapter 3

Menopause's revolutionary benefits

To address the peculiarity of how normal determination can lean toward the cessation of propagation, one must first provide the transformational benefit of menopause. To do this, four models of menopause are examined.

1. Its explicit species-level and hereditary nature

2. Its historical transformation

3. its unique value for human longevity

4. Its potential role in human development

A brief analysis of the wording reveals that the first two models are true. The third criterion is supported by research into four New Britain family histories, which revealed that among 1,890 women born between 1675 and 1874, those who died postmenopausally had better overall health than those who died before. The discovery that postmenopausal ladies also showed more notable ripeness could be used to address age-free improvement in endurance. In light of the belief that the presence of post-reproductive females who served as infant carriers would promote population growth through decreased birth division among mobile primate groups, a hypothesis for the genesis of menopause is advanced. As you approach the end of your fertile years, your body goes through menopause. You are not currently prepared to become pregnant when you reach menopause. Each woman uniquely experiences menopause, although it often begins when she is in her 40s or 50s. Several women believe that menopause is a sign that life is coming to an end. In any case, the average lifespan of a woman in the US is roughly 79 years, so you likely still have at least a portion of your life ahead of you.

It's common knowledge that menopause can have a wide range of terrible side effects. However, this typical organic transformation isn't entirely bad. Our team at OB/GYN Experts is now looking at a few usually disregarded benefits of menopause.

Elimination of women's periods

From adolescence until menopause, you have your monthly period. Throughout your lifetime, you typically experience about 500 of them. When you hit menopause, your ovaries stop making eggs. This ends your monthly cycle and the time between periods. There is no longer a strong incentive to buy tampons or pads, and there is no longer a chance of unexpected bleeding or spotting. and you are no longer able to become pregnant. That suggests to some women that they can have more enjoyable intercourse without worrying about an unplanned pregnancy.

Elimination of time-related incidentals

Your body undergoes hormonal changes as a result of your feminine cycle, which can have a variety of agonizing side effects for some women. When your periods stop, the hormonal changes also end. Nearly 90% of women experience premenstrual syndrome (PMS), and its negative effects include edema, crankiness, and migraines. In reality, feminine migraines affect over 60% of women with chronic headaches caused by cerebral discomfort. Before your period, your levels of estrogen and progesterone decline, which for some women causes pulsing head pain. If you have headaches during your regeneration years, you might notice that they stop after menopause since your chemical levels stop shifting permanently.

Reduced abdominal pain

Women in their reproductive years frequently protest by suffering from pelvic pain. The causes can include fibroids, ectopic pregnancies, and premature deliveries. When your period's stop, the pain associated with ovulation and heavy feminine emptying tightens. When estrogen levels are high, as they are during pregnancy and perimenopause, uterine fibroids—harmless growths—often develop. Fibroids can cause spotting and stomach torment, yet they start to disappear and side effects die down when you enter menopause.

A unique perspective

It's typical to experience a renewed sense of vitality in your postmenopausal years. In the 1950s, anthropologist Margaret Mead referred to this oddity as postmenopausal zing. Whether you realize it at the time or not, your monthly period is honestly and deeply taxing. Many women experience a newly discovered sense of sturdiness and confidence after being freed from the stress that comes with the conceptual years and coming on the other side of menopause. Women are more motivated to focus on themselves, creating plans to stock their lives, connections, and goals for the future. Research demonstrates that once you reach your 50s, optimistic thinking increases.

Chapter 4

Menopause's evolution

It is a privilege to mature. The changes to skin, hair, and chemicals that come along with it, however, frequently feel less dramatic. There is no avoiding the various effects of menopause, including drier skin, thinner hair, and decreased oil production. Nevertheless, despite being a normal part of life, "change" has been a topic shrouded in shame and mystery for a very long time.

Every woman will experience menopause since it is something that our bodies can do perfectly and naturally. The narrative that it is improper or shameful must end.

Menopause isn't discussed because of this tale, and most women leave this outing with little to no knowledge of what's happening and no assistance. Given that the vast majority of us have only heard horror stories, this fuels a lot of worries. Fortunately, the stigma around menopause is fading thanks to Gen Z's willingness to accept honesty regarding issues that are specifically relevant to women, such as periods and pregnancy.

Menopause is frequently mentioned as a whole, although it consists of three distinct stages: perimenopause, menopause, and post-menopause.

Menopause is the prolonged period when the female cycle stops. Post-menopause includes all of the years after menopause when the body adjusts to its new lower levels of progesterone and estrogen. Perimenopause can start four to five years before menopause when estrogen and progesterone levels start to decline and the body prepares to stop ovulating.

40+ years old: perimenopause

Although you will still have periods during perimenopause, they will become less regular and shorter until they completely stop. You might also start seeing physical changes at this time, such as weight gain, mood swings, disturbed sleep, hot flashes, night sweats, drier skin, and diminished charisma, all of which are typical symptoms of hormonal imbalance.

The Skin

The deterioration of estrogen, progesterone, and testosterone is reflected in the skin changes that occur throughout the perimenopausal stage. This occasionally manifests as adult skin irritation, increased reactivity, and skin dryness. Less collagen and glycosaminoglycans (GAGs, such as corrosive hyaluronic acid) are produced by the skin, which causes it to become thinner and less plump. Pay close attention to products and medications that will stimulate the production of collagen, lock in moisture, and animate your skin cells.

The Hair

Because of inherited, metabolic, hormonal, and environmental changes to the hair follicle as well as to the hair strand itself, aging has effects on the hair as well. Legitimate haircare products and in-salon medications can help to break this cycle, restore the health of the hair, and repair the fingernail skin so that it is protected from external aggressors.

50+ years old: menopause

The idea that menopause must be a horrible experience is untrue. Instead, think of it as a life-altering experience that marks the beginning of another chapter. Menopause is a significant adjustment for the body to go through, so it's not surprising that there are a few bumps along the way. However, if you understand what's happening and know how to support your body throughout, you may be able to minimize those blows and get a smoother ride.

The fallback Chemicals used in sex can alter our circadian rhythm and stress response, which can cause sleep problems, hot flashes, and behavioral abnormalities in certain people. Fortunately, this will stop after a while. However, managing your worry and restlessness in the interim will help speed up the process. The skin might become noticeably more skinny and rigid during menopause, giving it a slightly "raw" appearance. Crow's feet can develop when little variations develop around highly active facial muscles like the mouth and eyes.

The supporting fat stack of the face is rearranged as a result of estrogen deprivation, hastening the essential volume loss that is the hallmark of facial aging, such as listing. Women frequently look more exhausted, unhappy, or enraged due to volume misfortune, shrinking skin, and muscle overactivity. However, there are things you can do to help with the frightful skin around the eyes and neck with medications like platelet-rich plasma therapy (PRP), which involves re-infusing the skin with the healing components of your blood. Although restorative injectables may seem unsettling, a reputable skin expert will want to advise you on the most natural-looking outcome that enhances your greatest features.

Reduced estrogen levels might make skin seem drier and more delicate, necessitating more nourishment in the form of oils, ceramides, and boundary security products. Estrogen has a warm interaction with the skin and, before menopause, has a role in collagen and hyaluronic acid production, skin hydration, and blockage ability. Using a combination of dark cohosh, sage, choline, and chromium, healthy homegrown supplements help support menopause with staging. Other suitable improvements to incorporate into your daily schedule include those abundant in collagen, hyaluronic acid, and L-ascorbic acid. Menopausal women thrive on a diet that is strong in protein and low in carbohydrates. Remember that everyone's needs are different, so discuss any dietary adjustments with your doctor or a trusted professional.

60 years old: menopause

As our estrogen levels decline, this hormone will no longer be able to positively affect our mood, digestion, bone density, and muscle growth. Keep your spirits up by looking for happiness in different places. Maintain your social connections, engage in daily appreciation and reflection, pay attention to daily improvement, and nourish your body with foods that promote mental well-being and help prevent osteoporosis.

Post-menopausal women start to worry about osteoporosis. In the five to seven years following menopause, some women can lose up to 20% of their bone thickness, so focusing on maintaining thickness should be crucial.

If osteoporosis is a concern, regularly engaging in weight training and resistance training can also help to strengthen bones, as well as supplements including vitamin D, mineral K2, and magnesium. To help with relaxation and stress reduction, supportive exercises like walking and yoga are also advised during this time.

The new commonplace

There is no mystical number that can tell you exactly how long post-menopausal side effects take to fade or go completely, but be comforted that they will. Acclimating to your new normal can take time. No matter your age, it's important to incorporate quality skincare products and nutrients into your daily wellness routine. These include cell-reinforcing lotions and gels, sunscreen, and serums containing vitamin A and L-ascorbic acid. There are numerous available types. For the greatest results, it is best to have a professional skin specialist hold your hand along the journey.

Complexities of menopause
The lack of estrogen associated with menopause is linked to the concomitant medical disorders that become more prevalent as women get older. Following menopause, women are likely to experience:

Women are prone to developing heart and vein (cardiovascular) infections after menopause. When your estrogen levels fall, your risk of developing a cardiovascular infection rises. The leading cause of death for both men and women is coronary disease. Therefore, it's important to maintain a normal weight, engage in regular exercise, and eat a healthy diet. Consult your PCP for advice on the best ways to protect your heart, such as how to lower your cholesterol or reduce your circulatory strain if it is too high.

Osteoporosis. Due to this illness, bones become weak and brittle, increasing the risk of breaking. You may experience rapid bone thinning during the first few years following menopause, increasing your risk of osteoporosis. Osteoporotic postmenopausal women are especially vulnerable to hip, wrist, and spine fractures. Incontinence of the urine You may experience regular, abrupt, compelling urges to urinate, followed by an obligatory loss of urine (ask about incontinence), or a lack of urine with hacking, chuckling, or lifting as the elasticity of your urethra and vaginal tissues declines. You might experience urinary tract infections more frequently.

Exercises that strengthen the pelvic floor muscles and the use of a potent vaginal estrogen may help to relieve incontinence-related side effects. Menopausal urinary tract and vaginal alterations that can cause urinary incontinence may also be successfully treated with chemicals.

Sexual prowess. During intercourse, vaginal dryness brought on by decreased moisture production and loss of adaptability can be uncomfortable and mildly depleting. The decreased feeling may also impair your desire for sexual activity (moxie). Vaginal creams and greases with water bases may be beneficial. Many women find it helpful to use a nearby vaginal estrogen treatment, which comes in the form of a vaginal cream, tablet, or ring if a vaginal ointment isn't effective enough.

Gaining weight Since digestion returns to normal following menopause, many women gain weight during this time. To maintain your weight, you might need to eat less and exercise more.

The sexual changes that accompany menopause, such as vaginal dryness and a lack of sex drive, can be challenging to deal with. Additionally, you can discover that you detest sex and struggle to reach the climax. As long as it isn't difficult, regular sexual activity may help keep your vagina healthy by improving blood flow. It becomes hard for you to get pregnant once you reach menopause because your ovaries cease producing eggs. However, you are still susceptible to bodily illnesses. On the off chance that you're not in that mood with one person, use more secure sex drills.

Chapter 5

Hormone therapy

To alleviate menopause side effects, chemical therapy (HT) is used. Your decision to receive chemical treatment may be influenced by your age, family medical history, personal medical history, and the severity of your menopausal symptoms. Talk to your doctor about the benefits and risks of HT, the many forms of HT, and alternative elective options.

What exactly are progesterone and estrogen?

The ovaries of a woman produce the chemicals estrogen and progesterone, which plays a role in a variety of bodily functions, such as:

It thickens the uterus's protective layer, preparing it for potential egg implantation.

affects how your body uses calcium, a key nutrient for growing bones.

maintains healthy blood cholesterol levels.

keeps the vagina healthy.

helps prevent osteoporosis.

What reaction does progesterone have?

Progesterone plays a role in a variety of bodily functions, such as:

keeps up with your pregnancy and prepares your uterus for the implantation of a treated egg.

reduces the load on the heart.

Develops rest and temperament further.

Chemical therapy (HT)?

Your ovaries no longer produce excessive amounts of progesterone and estrogen. Retransition toward menopause Unpleasant side effects may result from changes in these chemical levels. Typical side effects of menopause include:

Glimmers of heat

There were night sweats and icy glimmers.

Dryness of the vagina; discomfort during sex

desire to urinate (urinary criticalness)

Snoozing is inconvenient (sleep deprivation)

Mood fluctuations, mild wretchedness, or grumpiness

Dry tongue, dry eyes, or dry skin

Your chemical levels are helped by chemical treatment (HT), which also relieves some menopausal adverse symptoms. Consult your healthcare provider about whether you should think about receiving HT treatment. Taking HT comes with a variety of health benefits and risks.

What types of chemical treatments (HT) are there?

The two most common types of chemical therapy (HT) are:

Treatment with estrogen: Estrogen is taken by itself. Most usually, doctors advise taking a fix or pill with a low estrogen content regularly. Additionally, estrogen may be suggested as a cream, vaginal ring, gel, or splash. To lessen the adverse effects of menopause and to prevent osteoporosis, you should consume the least amount of estrogen recommended.

Chemical treatment using estrogen, progesterone, and/or progestin (EPT): This type of HT, also known as a blend treatment, combines doses of estrogen and progesterone (or progestin, a manufactured type of progesterone).

What benefits come with receiving chemical therapy (HT)? It is advised to use chemical therapy

(HT) to lessen the negative effects of menopause, such as:

Smoky flames.

Dryness in the vaginal area may make sexual encounters challenging.

Menopause also comes with some challenging side effects, like night sweats and itchy, dry skin.

Additional health benefits of HT include:

decreased risk of developing osteoporosis and a reduced possibility of breaking a bone.

Enhanced mental health and a general sense of mental affluence in certain women.

Reduced teeth ill fortune

decreased the risk of colon disease

decreased the risk of diabetes

relief in joint pain that is subtle.

Women who undergo chemical treatment in their 50s have a lower mortality risk.

Chemical therapy (HT) is typically not advised in the following situations:

Have or ever had an endometrial illness or a cancerous tumor on the bosom?

Unusual vaginal death

possesses blood clusters or is at high risk for developing them.

Have a history of stroke, a coronary event, or an increased risk for vascular disease.

You may suspect or know you are pregnant.

The liver is infected.

What effects does chemical therapy (HT) have?

Chemical treatment has side effects, much like almost all other medications. The secondary effects that are most well-known include:

On the unlikely chance that you have a uterus and take cycled progestin (estrogen for 25 days of estrogen per month, progesterone for the last 10 to 14 days per month, and 3 to 6 days of no medication), you can experience month-to-month death.

Irregular spotting

Bosom treat.

Changes in mindset

More unusual outcomes of chemical processing include:

Liquid upkeep.

Brain aches (counting headache).

body stains (brown or dark spots).

The increased bosom thickness makes reading mammograms more challenging.

Skin irritation after estrogen treatment

How can I lessen these side effects of chemical therapy (HT)?

Typically, these side effects are mild and won't cause you to stop using HT. Obtain information about how to alter the type or measurement of the HT to lessen the adverse effects if your side effects annoy you. Never stop taking a medicine or adjust it without first consulting your doctor.

Chapter 6

Food plans for menopause

What constitutes a healthy menopause.

While menopause is associated with several uncomfortable side effects and increases your risk of certain illnesses, your food plan may help to lessen the adverse effects and speed up the process.

Variety of Foods to Eat

There is evidence that certain food types may help relieve some menopausal side symptoms, including hot flashes, poor sleep, and thin bones.

Dairy Goods

Women's risk of breakage can increase as a result of the decline in estrogen levels throughout menopause. Milk, yogurt, and cheddar are dairy products that include calcium, phosphorus, potassium, magnesium, and vitamins D and K, all of which are essential for healthy bones. In a study involving nearly 750 postmenopausal women, those who consumed more dairy and animal protein on average had thicker bones than those who consumed less of it. Dairy products may also help you get better sleep. According to a survey inquiry, menopausal women's sleep quality improved when they consumed foods high in the corrosive amino acid glycine, such as milk and cheddar. Additionally, research links dairy consumption to a lower risk of early menopause, which occurs before the age of 45. According to one study, women who consumed the most calcium and vitamin D, which are found in cheese and fortified milk, had a 17% lower risk of going through menopause early.

Firm Fats

Omega-3 unsaturated fats, which are solid, may benefit women going through menopause. Omega-3 supplements were believed to lessen the severity of night sweats and the frequency of hot flashes, according to a study of 483 menopausal women. However, in a separate analysis of 8 studies on omega-3 and menopausal side effects, a few studies supported the beneficial effect of unsaturated fat on hot flashes. Results were therefore unreliable. In light of everything, it very well may merit investigating to see if increasing your omega-3 intake worsens your menopause-related adverse effects. The foods that are highest in omega-3 unsaturated fats are found in fatty fish like mackerel, salmon, and anchovies, as well as seeds like flax, chia, and hemp.

Whole Grains

Whole grains are rich in vitamins and minerals, such as fiber and B vitamins including thiamine, niacin, riboflavin, and pantothenic acid. A diet rich in whole grains has been linked to a decreased risk of heart disease, cancer, and unanticipated losses.

In a study, researchers discovered that people who consumed at least three servings of whole grains daily had a 20–30% lower risk of developing diabetes and cardiovascular disease. Compared to people who typically consume refined carbohydrates, According to a study of more than 11,000 postmenopausal women, consuming 4.7 grams of whole grain fiber per 2,000 calories daily reduced the risk of dying young by 17% as opposed to eating only 1.3 grams per 2,000 calories. Whole grain food variations include quinoa, rye, whole wheat bread, grain, and rice with an earthy hue.

Soil-derived products

The byproducts of the soil are rich in fiber, minerals, and cell reinforcements. Therefore, according to American dietary guidelines, make a percentage of your plate out of green items. In a one-year mediation study including more than 17,000 menopausal women, those who consumed more veggies, natural products, fiber, and soy saw a 19% reduction in hot flashes compared to the control group. Healthier eating habits and weight loss were blamed for the drop. Cruciferous veggies may be especially beneficial for postmenopausal women. According to one study, consuming broccoli increased levels of an estrogen type that protects against the development of breast cancer while decreasing levels of an estrogen type linked to breast disease.

Dark berries may also be beneficial for menopausal women. In an eight-week study involving 60 menopausal women, 25 grams of freeze-dried strawberry powder per day decreased pulse when compared to the control group. In any case, additional research is necessary. In a second eight-week study with 91 moderately aged women, those who consumed 200 mg of daily grape seed extract supplements reported fewer hot flashes, better sleep, and reduced levels of sorrow compared to the control group.

foods that contain phytoestrogen.

Phytoestrogens are food-based intensifiers that act as weak estrogens in your body. While there has been some debate about including them in the diet, the most recent research suggests they may benefit well-being, particularly for women going through menopause. Soybeans, chickpeas, peanuts, flax seeds, grains, grapes, cherries, plums, green and dark tea, and a few more foods are typical sources of phytoestrogens. In a review of 21 studies on soy, postmenopausal women who took soy isoflavone supplements for about a month had 14% greater levels of estradiol (estrogen) than those who took a placebo. But the outcomes weren't very significant.

Suitable Protein

Reduced bone density and body mass are associated with the drop in estrogen that occurs with menopause. Therefore, menopausal women should consume more protein. According to rules, women over 50 should have 20–25 grams of high-quality protein every dinner, or 0.4–0.55 grams of protein per pound (1–1.2 grams per kg) of body weight, daily.

For all persons over the age of 18, the Recommended Dietary Allowance (RDA) for protein in the US is 0.36

grams per pound (0.8 grams per kilogram) of body weight, which is the bare minimum required for health. The range for protein in the recommended macronutrient distribution is 10–35% of the total daily calories.

In a recent study of 131 postmenopausal women over a year, those who consumed 5 grams of collagen peptides daily fared much better in terms of bone mineral density than those who consumed a powdered placebo. Your body has the highest concentration of collagen protein. Eating dairy protein was associated with an 8% lower risk of hip fracture in a large sample of persons over 50, whereas consuming plant protein was associated with a 12% lower risk.

Foods rich in protein include dairy items, eggs, meat, fish, and lentils. Protein powders can also be included in baked goods or smoothies.

Conclusion

Menopause, which is viewed as a sign of maturing, complicates the relationships between a woman's natural, social, and societal spheres. All of the women in the lifestyle shown have irregular menstrual cycles that cease in middle age. But women experience the emotional and social aspects of menopause in less common ways.

Clinical interventions that provide helpful indications continue to be a big aspect of treatment. However, the focus on biomedical concerns does not overshadow the social and mental expression of integrated social viewpoints toward development. The way of life is a source of imagery that people draw from to express their experiences. They are also concerned about their place in the cultural and societal structure as well as the interpersonal interactions between mothers and daughters and husbands and wives. One thing is certain: Many women welcome the end of reproduction as a relief to their bodies and a chance for new experiences, despite the obvious sign of age and the effect on identity.

www.ingramcontent.com/pod-product-compliance
Lightning Source LLC
Chambersburg PA
CBHW050316220526
45465CB00005B/2014